D1541121

God's Pathway
to Healing
PROSTATE

God's Pathway to Healing

PROSTATE

by

Reginald B. Cherry, M.D.

ALBURY PUBLISHING
Tulsa, Oklahoma

Note: The directions given in this book are in no way to be considered a substitute for consultation with your own physician.

God's Pathway to Healing Prostate
ISBN 1-57778-131-7
Copyright © 2000 by Reginald B. Cherry, M.D.
Reginald B. Cherry Ministries, Inc.
P. O. Box 27711
Houston, TX 77227-7711

Published by ALBURY PUBLISHING
P. O. Box 470406
Tulsa, Oklahoma 74147-0406

CONTENTS

INTRODUCTION

It strikes almost a quarter million men annually and will kill almost forty thousand men this year. It is now the most common cancer found in men and affects one man in eight.

It is prostate cancer.

Even more common is prostate enlargement (known as BPH, or Benign Prostatic Hyperplasia). Sixty percent of men between the ages of 60 and 70 have an enlarged prostate and 80 to 90 percent of men between 70 and 80 have enlargement in the prostate gland.

Traditional medicine has said that it is not *if,* but *when* a man will develop prostate problems—that if a man lives long enough, he will be attacked. As a believer, I do not accept this as inevitable. I believe that no weapon formed against us will prosper (see Isaiah 54:17). I also believe that God is revealing specific things in the natural that we can do to prevent, and even reverse, prostate disease.

Traditional treatments for the prostate are to "cut it, freeze it, burn it, or irradiate it," but fortunately we are advancing beyond these as our only options. Many prostate problems can be treated with natural supplements and compounds from the original plant kingdom God created for our food as mentioned in Genesis 1:29.

Are you familiar with plant-derived supplements such as saw palmetto, pygeum, beta-sitosterol, isoflavonoids, rye pollen, stinging nettle, and PC-SPES? Combinations of various natural treatments can benefit the symptoms of an enlarged prostate (difficulty starting urination, failure to empty the bladder completely, getting up frequently at night) and even provide benefit in those attacked with cancer of the prostate.

The Apostle Paul told us that we should not be unaware of the schemes or devices of the enemy (See 2 Corinthians 2:11). Therefore, it is important to get information about your body and have your prostate checked periodically. Men are particularly bad about dealing with attacks against their bodies, but in the case of the prostate, a simple blood test (a PSA test) and a digital exam (DRE) can yield critical information that can protect you from serious future problems. First and foremost it will show you how to pray specifically about the attack of the enemy. Then God may lead you to a simple natural supplement or food to deal with the problem, enabling you to avoid prescription medicines, surgery, or other procedures. Would you do something simple to protect this vital area of your body? Of course you would! All you need is good information and a revelation of what God would have you do in both the natural and the supernatural realms.

Medicine typically approaches prostate problems in a cookbook fashion. That is, doctors tend to treat every person the same way. This isn't strictly biblical, however, because in Psalm 139:14 David said that each of us is "fearfully and wonderfully made." This means that each of us is unique and each of us needs to seek God for our unique *Pathway to Healing*.

There are many reasons we can be attacked in areas such as the prostate. We can be disobedient to or ignorant of God's nutritional laws. In Exodus 23:25, God said His blessing was first on our bread and water (what we eat and drink) and *then* He would take disease from our midst. We will discuss the nutritional aspect of God's health laws and how they affect prostate disease.

It is also important for you to understand that being attacked in your body is not necessarily due to a lack of faith or being out of the will of God (it can be, but isn't always). The Bible says, "Many are the afflictions of the righteous: but the Lord delivereth him out of them all" (Psalm 34:19). We may not know why we were attacked, but we sure can know how to overcome the attack. Many righteous people are attacked in their bodies simply because they are such a threat to the kingdom of darkness that Satan attempts to cripple them with disease. God, however, will give revelation to the believer who remains under His umbrella of protection. He will reveal specifically how to resist and overcome the attack of the enemy. Remember, "Greater is he that is in you, than he that is in the world" (1 John 4:4).

God has specific ways for you to overcome and prevent prostate problems. These may or may not coincide with the strict protocols of modern medicine. But His ways are above our ways and His thoughts above our thoughts (see Isaiah 55:8-9).

Study the words of this book carefully and allow the Holy Spirit to give you specific wisdom and knowledge. Don't wait until you have symptoms of prostate problems. Start now. If you do have prostate problems or if you know someone who does, start down your *Pathway to Healing* today. Do what you can do in the natural and God will do what you can't do in the supernatural. God cares about you and His hand is reaching out to guide you down your *Pathway to Healing* prostate problems. He wants you to finish your course with joy!

Reginald B. Cherry, M.D.

Chapter 1

GOD HAS A PATHWAY TO HEALING FOR YOU

Chapter 1

GOD HAS A PATHWAY TO HEALING FOR YOU

Before we begin discussing prostate disease, how to pray for it, and what natural substances to take for it, I want to set the spiritual foundation for your healing.

As a medical doctor, I am keenly aware that I am only a helper in the healing process. Once I've diagnosed the likely cause of an illness, prescribed the appropriate medication or treatment, and explained the process to the patient, there is only one thing left to do. Actual healing is performed by God; I only treat. More than anyone else involved, I realize and acknowledge that the patient's manifestation of healing is dependent upon his faith in the Word of God and his obedience to God's natural health laws.

So what is the one thing left for me to do? I pray! In fact, I pray throughout the entire process—for inspiration, for revelation, for wisdom, for guidance, and for the manifestation of healing. I am part of a growing number of physicians who pray for and with their patients. With few exceptions, most patients want and appreciate prayer. It calms and reassures them. It drives out fear. It gives them hope and increases their faith to expect to be healed and to participate in the healing process.

But I pray very specifically. I pray, for example, for a patient's *Pathway to Healing*. This is based on the rather unique illustration of healing in Jesus' ministry cited in John, chapter 9. Jesus placed mud and saliva on the blind man's eyes, but the blind man was not healed. Jesus then instructed him to go down to the pool called Siloam, reach down in the water, and wash the mud away. In John 9:7, the Bible says that as he went his way and washed, he was healed. Thus God instructed me to set myself in agreement with each of my patients for their unique *Pathway to Healing*.

COMBINING THE NATURAL WITH THE SUPERNATURAL

I believe each person has a unique *Pathway to Healing* that involves both the supernatural as well as the natural, and God will reveal this unique pathway as we seek Him for it. I am thankful for the supernatural, instantaneous healings that occurred under Jesus' ministry. We should expect the same today. However, God's instruction to me has been to have people consider carefully that their healing may involve the combination of the natural with the supernatural. Really, all healing comes from God and thus is supernatural.

Proverbs 18:9 is one of the most astounding and eye-opening scriptures in the Bible. *The Amplified Bible* translates it: "He who does not use his endeavors to heal himself is brother to him who commits suicide." What an amazing insight God gave us in this scripture—pointing to the fact that the patient has a role to play in the pursuit of divine health through his own unique *Pathway to Healing!*

Our generation of physicians is just beginning to realize the limitations of modern medicine and is seeking information in the natural realm to help protect the health of our patients. Together, physicians and their patients are realizing that God has provided many natural pathways for us to help guard and protect our health.

This new focus in medicine is popularly called complementary or alternative medicine. When we study God's Word, however, we actually discover the ultimate form of complementary or alternative medicine: combining natural, God-created substances with the supernatural power of prayer to achieve healing and maintain health in our bodies.

As knowledge increases in these last days, I want to share with you the exciting information that God is revealing. I want to help you discover and walk down your unique *Pathway to Healing*, enabling you to combine your natural endeavors with your faith. You can combine the powerful anointing of the Holy Spirit, which resides within you as a child of God, with appropriate medical treatment and the utilization of various natural substances provided by our Creator for your benefit.

I realize more and more that the evil one, who is the source of all disease, is not so much interested in attacking our physical bodies as he is intent on striking at the "treasure [contained] in [our] earthen vessels" (2 Corinthians 4:7; inserts mine). The "treasure" he desires to hinder is the powerful, unstoppable anointing of God that resides in this earthen vessel, our physical body. If the enemy can cripple and disable our physical bodies, he can quench the anointing that is within and prevent us from going into all the world and being a light to that world (see Mark 16:15 and Matthew 5:14).

I have been able to watch many of my patients who were healed from a great many different diseases as they have learned to live by the principles that reveal God's *Pathway to Healing*. As they learned to identify His specific plan for them, learned to speak to their mountains of disease (see Mark 11:23-24), and commanded their mountains to fall in submission to God's plan, they found the healing they were so desperately seeking.

Yes, we would all like to be healed instantly, supernaturally, and miraculously. Thank God that miracles are still taking place. Jesus is the "same yesterday, and to day, and for ever" according to Hebrews 13:8. But, as we saw in John 9, sometimes we are healed as we go our way, following the instructions God has given us—and this path is no less supernatural. As you seek God for the specific pathway that will lead to your healing of prostate cancer or prostate enlargement, apply the principles you will learn in this book to your healing. Find a doctor who understands these principles and will pray in agreement with you.

WHAT CAUSES PROSTATE DISEASE?

Keep in mind that medically the cause of prostate cancer is still unknown. Research has suggested a combination of hormonal and genetic factors and perhaps dietary and environmental causes. What is clear is that early detection and improved treatments present men with important choices that may affect the length and quality of their lives.

The risk of prostate cancer increases with age. African-American men and men with a family history of prostate cancer (especially a father or brother) are also at greater risk. In its earliest stages, prostate cancer may not manifest any symptoms. Therefore, the most important thing is that your physician includes a Digital Rectal Examination (DRE) as part of your annual physical. You also should have a Prostate Specific Antigen (PSA) blood test every year. Again, if you're an African-American man or a man with a strong family history of prostate cancer, the PSA should be done annually, starting at age forty.

The PSA is a blood test that measures the amount of a protein, which is secreted into the blood by the prostate gland. Both normal and cancerous cells produce this antigen. Although some cancers produce PSA levels that measure in the normal range (0 to 4), most prostate cancers produce increased amounts of this antigen. A normal result does not exclude the presence of prostate cancer. But when the PSA is above normal, it suggests the possibility of prostate cancer.

Upon diagnosis, the course of treatment for prostate cancer is traditionally tailored to the stage (related to tumor size and whether it has spread beyond the prostate), the grade of the cancer (how fast the cancer is growing—some are slow-growing, others are aggressive), your age, your general health status, and the possible side effects of any treatment.

Age is a critically important consideration in treatment options. A physician may recommend no immediate treatment for a man of advanced age with prostate cancer that is slow growing, causing no symptoms, and is confined to the prostate gland. If the "watchful waiting approach" is chosen, the physician will closely monitor the size of the tumor, regularly test the PSA level, and proceed with appropriate treatment if the cancer begins to be life threatening.

But we're not going to take the "watchful waiting approach" that traditional physicians talk about. We are going to actively attack disease in our bodies with the power of prayer and with natural substances. Do not ever accept from a physician an approach that involves "watchful waiting." We are not going to accept anything the enemy is trying to bring on us!

Sometimes God does have us use traditional medical approaches. For a man in his fifties or sixties with a high-grade tumor, standard treatment will often extend his life. Improvements in nerve-sparing surgery and radiation therapy have reduced the risk of undesirable side effects. But as mentioned earlier, surgery and radiation are no longer considered the only forms of effective treatment. In the following chapters we will discuss God's *Pathway to Healing,* as well as preventing, prostate cancer and prostate enlargement through natural means.

YOU HAVE A PATHWAY TO HEALING PROSTATE DISEASE

The most important thing for you to keep in mind is that God has a pathway for the manifestation of your healing to take place. Philippians 4:19 reminds us that "God shall supply all your need according to his riches in glory by Christ Jesus." If you—or someone you know—

have need of healing for prostate disease, whether prostate enlargement or prostate cancer, God has provided you with ways to pray specifically and with understanding about the prostate.

Above all, know that the price for your healing has already been paid in full! Let your hope soar and your faith increase as you wait expectantly for the manifestation of your healing of prostate disease. Join me in seeking some insights God has given, so that we men can be set free from the symptoms and diseases relative to the prostate.

Chapter 2

GOD'S PATHWAY TO HEALING PROSTATE ENLARGEMENT

Chapter 2

GOD'S PATHWAY TO HEALING PROSTATE ENLARGEMENT

Enlargement of the prostate gland is by far the most common prostate problem men will face. Prostate enlargement (or BPH) is benign, but it can cause a lot of misery. It is not cancer and does not turn into cancer (though a man can have both BPH and prostate cancer at the same time). This condition is typically found in men over 45. Recent statistics I've seen show that roughly 60 percent of men between the ages of 60 and 70 have an enlarged prostate,[1] with the percentage approaching 80 to 90 percent in men between the ages of 70 and 80.[2]

How can one little gland cause so many difficulties? The problem is its location. The urethra, which carries urine from the bladder to the outside of the body, runs right through the middle of this gland and when it gets larger, problems can occur with the flow of urine from the bladder. In severe cases prostate enlargement can shut off the flow of urine completely, which is a medical emergency.

WHAT IS THE PROSTATE?

What is the prostate and what is it for? Well, basically the prostate makes it possible for the human race to reproduce itself. The prostate makes it possible for a male to father children. Sperm are not produced in the prostate, but are produced in the testicles. The prostate, however, secretes a fluid (seminal fluid) that transports the sperm. Sperm are very fragile. The seminal fluid from the prostate helps nourish these fragile sperm and also helps make the vaginal canal acidic. These factors all must come together for an ovary to be fertilized and a woman to conceive.

The prostate starts off pretty small. At birth it is about the size of an almond and remains this size throughout early childhood. During a male's teen years, however, the prostate begins to increase in size until it approximately doubles. This is in preparation for sexual reproduction. The testicles begin producing sperm and the seminal fluid is produced by the prostate to nourish and support the sperm.

Everything works fine until a male reaches age forty-five to fifty. Then the prostate starts growing again. It is this second growth spurt that causes problems. In some men it continues enlarging for the rest of their lives. In others it only enlarges slightly and then stops. As we will see, the nutrients a man takes into his body can have a profound effect on whether the prostate keeps getting bigger or stops growing.

SYMPTOMS OF PROSTATE ENLARGEMENT

The growth spurt in middle age is generally felt to be influenced by hormonal changes in a man's body. As we have seen, the urethra runs right through the middle of the prostate. As the prostate gland enlarges and begins to squeeze the urethra, the normal flow of urine is affected and uncomfortable symptoms begin occurring. As the urethra is squeezed by the prostate enlargement, the bladder has to contract harder and harder as it tries to push urine out of the body, and the wall of the bladder can actually thicken. If the prostate continues to enlarge, the bladder has to work even harder to force urine through the narrowed urethra and it gets more and more sensitive, which can result in an almost continual urge to urinate. One of the first symptoms a man notices as the prostate enlarges is getting up more frequently during the night, and secondly a continuing sense of urgency or sudden uncontrollable urge to urinate.

Here is a checklist of symptoms for an enlarged prostate:

_____ Need to urinate frequently, especially during the night

_____ Sudden uncontrollable urge to urinate

_____ Weak or interrupted urine flow

_____ Inability to urinate (difficulty starting or stopping)

_____ Burning sensation or pain when urinating

_____ Blood in urine

_____ Reduced sexual ability

_____ Discomfort during intercourse

WHY DOES THE PROSTATE ENLARGE?

Most current research indicates a hormonal imbalance causes prostate enlargement. Just as women's hormones change during menopause, so too do men's hormones change. As men get older, the levels of the male hormone (testosterone) gradually decrease while men's estrogen levels increase (yes, men do produce estrogen just as women produce testosterone). The testosterone levels that remain are converted into higher levels of the active form known as DHT (dihydrotestosterone). It is increasing levels of DHT that also contribute to baldness in aging men if they have the genetic susceptibility. These higher levels of DHT and increased estrogen stimulate the prostate gland to increase in size.

One of the keys, then, to preventing (and reversing) enlargement of the prostate is to prevent testosterone from being converted into its more active DHT form. There is an enzyme within the prostate called 5-alpha-reductase that performs this conversion. Many of the natural treatments for prostate enlargement work by inhibiting this enzyme. This is how saw palmetto works, which we will discuss in a moment.

Remember, if you're having any of the symptoms mentioned previously, don't try to make a diagnosis yourself. Consult with a knowledgeable physician. Many of these symptoms can also be indicative of prostate cancer, and you must know what the attack of the enemy is to effectively overcome it. Remember too that many doctors can make an accurate diagnosis, but they also like to do surgery or use prescription drugs to treat the problem. American men spend over three billion dollars yearly on prostate surgery. While cutting out the enlarged prostate tissue can be effective in alleviating symptoms, it can also cause impotence and incontinence (leakage of urine from the bladder). Let's look at some of the natural options first.

NATURAL REMEDIES

Saw Palmetto. Probably the most popular and one of the most effective natural treatments is the herb saw palmetto *(Serenoa repens)*. It is the extract of the saw palmetto berry that is so effective for the prostate. The saw palmetto extract inhibits the 5-alpha-reductase enzyme, which in turn lowers the amounts of the potent DHT form of testosterone. This is exactly the way the expensive prescription drug *Proscar* works. This plant from God's natural

creation, however, has several more benefits than man's synthetic drug. Saw palmetto has anti-inflammatory properties,
which decrease inflammation within the
prostate gland itself. It also contains beta
sitosterol, which has anti-inflammatory
properties and also strengthens the
body's immune system. Over eighteen
published studies involving more than
twenty-nine hundred men have shown
significant improvement in symptoms as
well as peak urinary flow. These studies
have been reported in the prestigious
medical journal, *JAMA*.[3] The usual dose
of saw palmetto is 160 mg. twice daily,
utilizing an 85 to 95 percent free-fatty-
acid standardized extract. Note that it
can take from a few weeks up to as long

as three months for the saw palmetto to exert its beneficial effects. It can, however, be taken indefinitely with no long-term side effects.

Pygeum. Pygeum (also known as the African plum tree) has shown some remarkable effects in reducing the symptoms of prostate enlargement. Pygeum is an evergreen tree that grows in Africa. An extract from the bark of this tree has been utilized in Europe for several decades and found quite effective at improving urinary flow, stopping the urgency of urination, and decreasing inflammation in the prostate. It is often combined with saw palmetto and in many ways works similar to saw palmetto, though some herbalists feel it is even stronger than the saw palmetto extract. It blocks the effects of the male hormone testosterone on the prostate gland and also contains beta sitosterol, which is very effective for prostate health. The typical dose of pygeum is 50 to 100 mg. twice daily.

South African Stargrass. A recent medical journal article reported that an extract from South African stargrass, which contains mainly beta sitosterol, showed a significant effect in shrinking the prostate gland and relieving symptoms. Marketed in Germany as *Harzol* and *Azuprostat,* studies are showing very promising results from these preparations and extracts that are high in beta sitosterol. Exact dosages and amounts vary, but in this situation you would need to follow the instructions on the label.

Stinging Nettle. In Germany extracts from the roots of the stinging nettle plant *(Urtica dioica)* have been used to effectively treat prostatic enlargement. Who would think that God would use a plant known as "stinging nettle" to help relieve prostate symptoms?! The root of the stinging nettle contains many of the active ingredients in saw palmetto. It appears to have even more prominent anti-inflammatory properties. The extract contains sterols, lignans, lectins, and phenols. Typically the stinging nettle extract is added to either saw palmetto or pygeum rather than being used alone.

A typical dosage should be 300 to 600 mg. of the root daily.

Rye Pollen. In Europe, pollen extracts are marketed under the name *Cernilton*. In particular, an extract from rye pollen contains several water soluble and fat soluble compounds that increase the force of contraction of the bladder muscle (the detrusor muscle) and also inhibit the 5-alpha-reductase enzyme, which in turn helps shrink the prostate's size. In a study in Japan utilizing rye pollen extract *(Cernilton),* 50 percent of the men reported excellent results and improvement of urinary symptoms. The dosage used in the study was 126 mg. three times daily, with no side effects recorded.[4]

Red Clover Plant Extracts. Also known as isoflavones, red clover plant extracts have had excellent results in treating the symptoms associated with a prostate enlargement. A single 40-mg. tablet daily (marketed under the brand name *Trinovin)* resulted in a 21 percent reduction in symptoms after only thirty days, and an average 30 percent reduction in symptoms after three months. The most significant benefit of the red clover extract was decreasing the need for men to urinate during the night. Also, red clover extracts appear to have a more rapid onset of action than some of the other herbal treatments. These results were reported in a presentation based on research at the University of

Chicago as well as the Columbia University College of Physicians and Surgeons.[5] The red clover extract contains four different isoflavones: genistein, daidzein, biochanin, and formononetin. These work by inhibiting the conversion of testosterone to DHT, and they also prevent the effects of increased estrogen levels on the prostate as we talked about earlier. These red clover extracts are very safe and taking one 40-mg. tablet daily has produced excellent results.

Genistein. A major isoflavone found in soy products, genistein has also been shown to have a positive effect on decreasing the growth of human prostate tissue. It tends to block the estrogen receptors, which in turn renders the estrogen less active in causing prostate enlargement. A simple way to aid prostate health would be to add a soy product, such as eight ounces of soymilk or a soy protein, to our daily diet. In Europe they have even developed a soy cookie which is intended to promote prostate health. It's very interesting that in Asia, where genistein and soy products are consumed in much higher amounts, the incidence of prostate enlargement (and prostate cancer) is much lower. This is probably related to their diet, and soy appears to be a significant component of this beneficial diet.

God has blessed us with many compounds, which we are only now beginning to understand, to help with the common problem of prostate enlargement. Before you allow your prostate to be "cut, burned, vaporized, or microwaved," try the natural route!

Chapter 3

GOD'S PATHWAY
TO HEALING
PROSTATE CANCER

Chapter 3

GOD'S PATHWAY
TO HEALING
PROSTATE CANCER

Though prostate cancer is the most common cancer in men, it is not quite the deadliest. Approximately 100,000 men will be diagnosed with respiratory cancer this year and about 94,000 will die of the disease. Estimates vary, but approximately 180,000 men will be diagnosed with prostate cancer in this same period and over 31,000 will die of the disease.[1] This statistic tells us that many cases of prostate cancer are slow growing, and with a few simple steps many men who have been diagnosed with prostate cancer will live a long life and will not suffer any effects from it. Unfortunately, a majority of men are still not aware of this potential threat. Moreover, they do not understand that God has revealed a pathway to prevent and even treat this devastating disease with newer natural treatments.

GETTING YOUR PROSTATE CHECKED

It is important that men be checked on a regular basis with two tests for their prostate: the PSA and the DRE. The

Prostate Specific Antigen (PSA) blood screening should be done on all men over age 50 and on men under age 50 with a family history of prostate cancer. Prostate specific antigen is an enzyme made by prostate tissue that dissolves the proteins which cause semen to clump. Levels can be checked using a simple blood test. Elevated amounts of PSA may mean prostate cancer, although levels can increase due to age, sexual activity, and a variety of factors other than cancer.

For decades, diagnosis of prostate cancer relied upon a doctor's experience and ability to detect prostate abnormalities using just a finger during a digital rectal examination (DRE). The DRE remains a key test for prostate cancer. However, PSA screening and ultrasound imaging, which painlessly creates a picture of the prostate using sound waves, are helping physicians detect prostate cancer early enough to potentially cure it, while keeping adverse effects to a minimum.

PROSTATE CANCER PREVENTION

All men should follow the eight steps listed below to help prevent cancer from forming or to help cure it if it has been diagnosed. These alternatives to the traditional ways we practice medicine have been substantiated in numerous medical studies.

In Exodus 23:25, God said He would take disease from our midst, but first His blessing had to be on our food. With this in mind, these eight practical steps are part of God's pathway to your healing.

1. *Decrease Saturated Fat*—Eat beef no more than three times per month. Limit cheese and switch to skimmed milk or, even better, soymilk.

2. *Antioxidants*—Get plenty of vitamins C and E, beta-carotene from yellow, orange, and dark green fruits and vegetables, and selenium. Almonds (10 per day) can supply vitamin E. Add supplements: C (1,000 mg. twice daily), E (800 i.u. daily), beta-carotene (20,000 i.u. daily), and selenium (200 mcg. daily).

3. *Calcium*—Calcium can decrease the formation of tumor cells and may decrease the uptake of a fatty acid that

contributes to tumor formation (alpha linoleic acid). You should obtain calcium from non-fat yogurt, non-fat cottage cheese, and skimmed milk or soymilk. Also add a 1,000-mg. daily supplement of calcium in the form of calcium citrate, calcium ascorbate, and calcium carbonate.

4. *Garlic*—Garlic can limit tumor growth, kill cancer cells, and even shrink existing tumors. If you are at a high risk for developing prostate cancer or you have been diagnosed with prostate cancer already, I would suggest taking a garlic capsule equivalent to one clove of fresh garlic daily.

5. *Vitamin D*—Higher levels of vitamin D offer protection from prostate

cancer. Men in sunnier climates have a lower incidence of prostate cancer (sun causes the skin to make vitamin D). Don't overdo sun exposure; only fifteen minutes daily will produce protective amounts of vitamin D from your skin. Good sources from the diet include fish and skimmed milk. A daily supplement of 400 i.u. of vitamin D (cholecalciferol) will give you added insurance.

6. *Tea*—Compounds in green tea (catechins) can inhibit tumor growth. Again, if you are at high risk for prostate cancer or have been diagnosed with prostate cancer, drink two to four cups of green tea daily. We now also recommend green-tea extract in a

daily nutrient supplement because of its potent cancer-fighting effects throughout the body.

7. *Soy*—Soy products limit the spread of cancer and can even stop its early growth. Soymilk and soy flour are sources of this protective food. Another option is to use soy protein isolate powder.

8. *Cumin*—This spice, which can be used on vegetables and in various dishes, may prevent the development of prostate cancer.

DIET AND PROSTATE CANCER

Studies have revealed differences in the risk of prostate cancer among different populations worldwide. For example, the mortality rate for prostate cancer in the United States is more than 400 percent that of Japan. And the incidence of the disease in North America is 50 times higher than in China. But men in Japan or China who relocate to the United States acquire the higher risks of American men after only one or two generations, which tells us that it isn't just genetic.

Researchers suspect that diet—and the amount of dietary fat—is responsible. These men bring their families to "the land of plenty," and their rate of prostate cancer goes up 20 percent because they adopt our saturated-fat-filled diet. Saturated fat is number one on the list of reasons why American men are being affected by this increasingly common disease. We must reduce our intake of saturated fat. This translates to significantly decreasing our consumption of beef, cheese, and whole milk.

The American diet, with its high saturated fat consumption, is obviously one major culprit in increasing prostate cancer. Scientists at Harvard Medical School and the Harvard School of Public Health evaluated the diets of more than 50,000 health professionals over a four-year period. They found that the men who ate the most fat were nearly twice as likely to develop prostate cancer as men who ate the least fat. Men who ate the most beef, bacon, pork, and lamb were more than two-and-a-half times more likely to develop prostate cancer than the men who ate the least.[2]

Whole milk is another enemy of the prostate gland. Two glasses of whole milk weekly compared with one glass a week *doubles* the risk of prostate cancer! It's not the milk—it's the fat in the milk. Obviously, the same goes for cheeses. Fortunately, many fat-free cheeses are on the market now that are made from skimmed milk. So cheese isn't as great an issue as it once was, but we still need to monitor the saturated fat content. There are soymilks available which are very low in fat, offer significant prostate protection, and even taste good! (I know many of you are turning up your noses, but try it!) Soy is nondairy but has significant amounts of added calcium and other nutrients.

Our greatest protection from prostate cancer comes from substances derived from Genesis 1:29 where God originally gave us fruits and vegetables (herbs) and the seeds that they contain. In a recent study in the *Journal of the National Cancer Institute* men who ate three or more servings of cruciferous vegetables (broccoli, cauliflower, cabbage) had 41 percent lower risk of prostate cancer compared to men who ate less that one serving daily. Cruciferous vegetables stood out as being especially protective of prostate cancer.[3]

Broccoli and cauliflower, along with brussel sprouts and kale, showed the greatest preventive benefits. Fortunately with the new technology available in nutrient supplements, we can take extracts of broccoli and cauliflower—and all of the protective fruits and vegetables— and consume them daily along with our vitamins. There will be more on this later in this book.

LYCOPENE IN YOUR TOMATO

Research consistently indicates that tomatoes, especially cooked tomatoes or tomato paste, are protective against prostate cancer. Tomatoes contain many nutrients, among them vitamins C and B-complex and the minerals iron and potassium. Also in the mix are carotenoids. These include lycopene and beta-carotene, which is converted in the body into vitamin A.

Lycopene gets high marks from researchers for its apparently potent antioxidant properties. Antioxidants are thought to neutralize harmful "free radicals." These molecules, which result from normal cell metabolism as well as other causes, may contribute to cancer and cardiovascular disease.

A six-year study of approximately 48,000 men found that those eating ten servings of cooked-tomato products a week had the lowest risk of prostate cancer. A serving is equivalent to a half-cup of tomato or spaghetti sauce, a quarter cup of tomato paste, one medium tomato, or one slice of low-fat pizza with tomato sauce. The risk of advanced prostate cancer for those using tomato products was about one third that of men eating less than two servings a week.[4]

Fresh tomatoes are loaded with lycopene, but cooking tomatoes makes lycopene easier for your body to use. For instance, there is five times more available lycopene in tomato sauce than in an equivalent amount of fresh tomatoes. Apparently, heat breaks down tomato-cell walls, freeing lycopene that would otherwise pass through your digestive system. Also, including a little monounsaturated fat such as olive oil can improve absorption of lycopene.

Lycopene has proven to be such a powerful cancer fighter (even fighting breast cancer in women) that we have included it in our basic daily nutrient supplement. God has given us the ability to get the benefit of fruits and vegetables containing such potent substances as lycopene each day, even though we might not be able to consume all of them daily in our diets.

PROSTATE CANCER AND GREEN TEA

Researchers have known for years that the incidence of prostate cancer is considerably lower in Asian countries. One possible explanation advanced by scientists is the high consumption of plant foods among Asian populations. Another is the growing number of laboratory studies indicating that green tea—the most popular tea in China, Japan, and other Asian countries—has anti-tumor effects. The compounds in this tea affect not only prostate, but some research indicates that it inhibits the growth of skin cancer, esophageal cancer, and other internal cancers.

Americans typically consume black tea (which is a fermented tea). It is weaker and less potent, though it does have some of the same effects of green tea, which is not fermented. Lipton, the huge tea manufacturer, has now added green tea to its product line, so it is readily available in grocery stores. Green tea contains more chemicals that act as antioxidants and nontoxic, cancer-preventive agents than black tea. It has been speculated that the low lung-cancer rate in Japan—despite the high rate of smoking—is due to green tea consumption.

Green-tea extracts (catechins) are now available, so that we can ingest them daily along with our other vitamin, mineral, and nutrient supplements. I have found the research to be so impressive on green tea that I have incorporated it in our recommended daily nutrient supplements.

THE MEDITERRANEAN DIET

Vitamin and other nutritional deficiencies accumulate in our bodies over time—often the result of consuming too many refined foods, fats, sugars, etc., and eating too few fresh foods and too little fiber. To correct this problem, proper nutrition and vitamin, mineral, and herbal supplements should be the main focus of any changes you make to regain and maintain optimum prostate health, but they must be the right foods and supplements for your body.

Scientists have studied various diets around the world for several years. They have found that the Mediterranean diet is at the top of the list in terms of providing health benefits. Some of the lowest rates of heart disease and cancer recorded in the world have been noted in those countries around the eastern Mediterranean. It is believed that their unusually good health is related in large part to the nutritional consistency of their dietary intake. I urge you to study the basic outline of the Mediterranean diet and incorporate as many of these principles into your own diet as possible.

The Mediterranean diet contains many of the foods rich in the vitamins and minerals needed for consumption. We highly recommend this diet, which closely corresponds to Genesis 1:29 and 9:3.

The Mediterranean diet incorporates the following foods:

1. **Olive Oil.** Replaces most fats, oils, butter, and margarine. Use it in salads or cook with it. Olive oil raises the level of good cholesterol (HDL) and may strengthen immune system function. Extra virgin oil is preferable.

2. **Bread.** Consume daily, not sliced white bread or even sliced wheat bread, but dark, chewy, crusty loaves. Ezekiel bread (see Ezekiel 4:9) would be excellent.

3. **Pasta, Rice, Couscous, Bulgar, and Potatoes.** Pasta is often served with fresh vegetables and herbs sautéed in olive oil, occasionally with very small quantities of lean beef. Dark rice is preferred. Couscous and bulgar are forms of wheat.

4. **Grains.** Alternate cereals such as wheat bran ($1/2$ cup), Bran Buds ($1/2$ cup), or oat bran ($1/3$ cup) 4-5 times weekly.

5. **Fruit.** Preferably raw, 2-3 pieces daily.

6. **Beans.** Pintos, great northern, navy, and kidney ($^1/_2$ cup) 3-4 times weekly. Bean and lentil soups are very popular (with a small amount of olive oil).

7. **Nuts.** Almonds (10 per day) or walnuts (10 per day) are at the top of the list.

8. **Vegetables.** Dark green vegetables are prominent, especially in salads. Eat at least one of these daily: cabbage, broccoli, cauliflower, turnip greens, or mustard greens; and one of these daily: carrots, spinach, sweet potatoes, cantaloupe, peaches, or apricots.

9. **Cheese and Yogurt.** In the Mediterranean diet, cheese may be grated on soups or a small wedge may be served combined with a piece of

fruit for dessert. Use the reduced-fat varieties (the fat-free often tastes like rubber). The best yogurt is fat-free, but not frozen.

You should consume the following foods only a few times weekly:

10. **Fish.** The healthiest are cold-water varieties: cod, salmon, and mackerel. Trout is also good. All these are high in omega-3 fatty acids. Salmon is an excellent source of calcium.

11. **Poultry.** Can be eaten 2-3 times weekly. White breast meat is best. Remove skin.

12. **Eggs.** Eat in small amounts 2-3 times weekly.

Consume the following an average of three times per month:

13. **Red Meat.** Eat red meat no more than three times a month, and then only use lean cuts with fat trimmed. It should be no larger than the size of a deck of cards. It can also be used in small amounts to "spice up" soup or pasta. The severe restriction of red meat in the Mediterranean diet is a radical departure from the American diet and is a major contributor to the low cancer and heart disease rates in these countries.

Typically, a Mediterranean meal would consist of:

1. **Salad.** Eaten with each meal. Fresh greens and other vegetables with olive oil, vinegar, and/or lemon juice.

2. **Soup.** Often with chopped celery, garlic, carrots, or onions (sometimes in a chicken stock), with added herbs and a small amount of grated cheese (use low fat).

3. **Pasta.** A staple of many meals, often made with fresh vegetables and herbs sautéed in olive oil, occasionally a bit of beef or chicken is added.

4. **Rice.** Prominent in this diet and includes dark rice, pilafs, etc.

5. **Breakfast.** Often dark bread or cereal (such as those previously mentioned), a piece of fresh fruit, and perhaps a small amount of yogurt or a slice of low- or fat-free cheese.

6. **Tomatoes, Onions, Lemon Juice.** All common in the Mediterranean diet.

SUPPLEMENTS CAN PREVENT PROSTATE CANCER

There are four antioxidant supplements that are critical in the prevention of prostate cancer: vitamin C, E, beta-carotene, and selenium. I now recommend that all male patients supplement their diet in order to get extra amounts of these important substances. I recommend 1,000 mg. of vitamin C, twice daily, along with 800 i.u. of the natural form of vitamin E. The word *natural* should appear on the label. Chemically this is more potent than the synthetic (dl-alpha form). I also recommend 20,000 units of beta-carotene daily.

One of the most potent combinations that has turned up in research studies relating to the prevention of prostate cancer is the combination of vitamin E and the mineral selenium. Selenium functions as an antioxidant in the body and we recommend 200 mcg. of selenium (selenomethionine) daily. Taking a simple combination of vitamin E and selenium in the amounts noted have reduced the incidence of prostate cancer up to 50 percent in some studies.

Would you do something simple? Sure you would. All you need is good information and the willingness and desire to submit to the leading of the Holy Spirit to protect your temple.

CALCIUM SUPPLEMENTS FOR MEN?

This is interesting news because doctors have not traditionally promoted the benefits of calcium for men. We have always recommended that women take calcium to protect their bones from osteoporosis, but it has recently been determined that men can also protect their bones from similar calcium loss. Calcium can help lower blood pressure and prevent the formation of polyps in the colon, which lead to colon cancer. Some studies have suggested that 1000 mg. of calcium a day may decrease the uptake of certain types of fatty acids that may adversely affect the prostate. Other more recent studies, however, have indicated that taking high amounts of calcium can actually increase prostate cancer. Further analysis of this data indicates that it is probably not the calcium intake, but the fact that men who take high amounts of calcium without increasing their vitamin D intake are the ones at risk of increasing prostate cancer. Calcium must be taken along with supplemental vitamin D in the appropriate balance as calcium tends to decrease blood levels of vitamin D. Vitamin D is a known protector from prostate cancer.

I recommend taking 1000 mg. of calcium daily in divided doses in the form of citrate, gluconate, ascorbate, and carbonate combination simply because it appears in multiple forms in the foods we eat. The calcium, however, should be taken along with vitamin D in a balanced nutrient supplement. The appropriate dose of vitamin D (cholecalciferol) is 400 I.U. daily. Be careful about exceeding this amount, however, as excessive levels of vitamin D can have a toxic effect. The benefits of calcium are substantial and we now recommend that men as well as women take calcium in the proper dosage, form, and balanced with other nutrients.

GARLIC AND PROSTATE CANCER

Various studies have demonstrated that garlic actually has a destructive effect on abnormal tumor cells. Research has indicated that within two days of exposing abnormal prostate tumor cells to garlic, the tumor growth markedly diminishes. When purchasing a garlic supplement, it is important to be certain the label states the dosage is equivalent to one clove of garlic. I recommend taking this amount daily.

DECREASED SUNSHINE— MORE PROSTATE CANCER

The rate of prostate cancer increases in latitudes farthest from the equator. In other words, where there is less direct light from the sun, the potential for prostate cancer is greater. It is not the sunlight however, but the vitamin D it produces that protects men from prostate cancer.

On exposure to sunlight, the skin on the human body makes vitamin D, so the vitamin D in people who live closer to the equator is higher because of their exposure to the sun. They make more vitamin D and have less prostate cancer. But there is also a negative side to this truth.

Some people might get the idea that sunbathing for an hour or two a day will help prevent prostate cancer. But becoming a sun worshiper increases the risk of melanoma, keratosis, and other malignant skin diseases. As little as fifteen to twenty minutes a day produces all the vitamin D you need.

Skimmed milk is also fortified with vitamin D, along with cold-water fish like salmon, tuna, cod, mackerel, sea trout, and herring. Vitamin D is a cell regulator. It keeps the machinery that reproduces cells in the prostate from going out of control and turning into cancer. This supplement, however, must be limited to no more than 400 i.u. daily. Excessive amounts of vitamin D can cause toxic reactions.

HERB COMBINATION FOR PROSTATE CANCER

There has been a lot of stirring in prostate cancer research circles about a unique eight-herb combination known as PC-SPES. Men with advanced stages of prostate cancers have noticed dramatic drops in their PSA levels (which is an indicator of cancer activity; in general the higher the PSA, the greater the cancer spread and cancer volume in the body). In fact in some studies, 60 percent of men taking the PC-SPES supplement had undetectable levels of the PSA. More importantly, the men noticed a marked difference in their body and the way they felt.

Numerous clinical trials are underway on this non-prescription, over-the-counter supplement. Preliminary data indicates significant declines in the PSA level of more than 50 percent and as high as 60 percent of the men responding had undetectable PSA levels.

What is PC-SPES? It is a natural herbal combination that includes a specific form of ginseng, saw palmetto, and other less-familiar herbs. How do these plant substances created by God offer us a tool to fight prostate cancer? A recent report published in the *New England Journal of Medicine* indicated that the eight-herb combination has estrogenic activity, and the herbs also shut down the production of the male hormone testosterone.[5] This particular type of estrogenic activity may be acting on the estrogen receptors on prostate cancer cells, literally causing the cells to kill themselves.

Additional studies have found that PC-SPES slowed the growth of two distinct prostate cancer cell lines, which means it is inhibiting the growth of these abnormal cancer cells. Other studies indicate the herbs strengthen the body's immune system and reduce the activity of a cancer gene known as Bcl-2.

Clearly there is something going on with this herbal combination that is beneficial. It is lowering PSA levels in many men with advanced prostate cancer and, more importantly, it is improving their overall quality of life by controlling the cancer.

There are some annoying side effects from this potent herb combination, though, due to drops in testosterone levels. Decreased libido, hot flashes, and leg cramps have been reported. You should be under the care of a knowledgeable physician who is familiar with this product if you use it. We will keep our ministry partners posted in our monthly newsletter, *Pathway to Healing,* as the latest studies on PC-SPES become available.

RISK FACTORS FOR
PROSTATE CANCER DEVELOPMENT

It is well established that the incidence of prostate cancer advances with increasing age. While it is a very unusual disease in men before age 50, rates increase exponentially thereafter. And it does tend to run in families. Approximately 15 percent of men with a diagnosis of prostate cancer will be found to have had a first-generation male relative (a brother or father) with prostate cancer, compared to approximately 8 percent of the general U. S. population.

Many men have prostate cancer for years without being aware of their condition. The cancer often grows slowly, remains within the prostate, and causes no problems. It can, however, spread rapidly, aggressively, and cause death. Even when prostate cancer is identified through a biopsy, it's difficult to accurately predict whether it will be life threatening or not, though progress is being made in this area.

THE PROSTATE CHECKLIST

Are you a candidate for prostate disease? Check any of the symptoms listed below that you might be experiencing now. If three or more of these symptoms describe your physical condition, you should consult with a knowledgeable physician to discuss treatment for prostate disease:

_____ Pain and/or difficulty in urinating (slow or sluggish emptying of bladder)

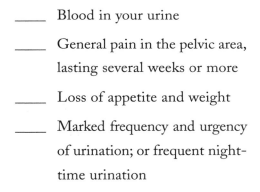

_____ Blood in your urine

_____ General pain in the pelvic area, lasting several weeks or more

_____ Loss of appetite and weight

_____ Marked frequency and urgency of urination; or frequent night-time urination

TRADITIONAL TREATMENTS FOR PROSTATE CANCER

All of the evidence that we have just shared with you points to the simple fact that God does indeed have a plan to protect men from prostate cancer and prostate enlargement. Is there something to the fact that Asian men don't suffer from the symptoms of this disease as much as American men? Are the studies coming out of prestigious research centers regarding natural substances simply confirming God's original plan? Yes, I believe God is revealing something to our generation that we are just beginning to grasp. Most importantly, He is making it easy for us to protect our bodies by not only giving us revelation knowledge, but also giving us the ability to use these substances every day in our busy lifestyles.

There are times, of course, when traditional medical treatment options are used for prostate cancer, and you simply have to seek God and follow peace concerning these. In any case, you should utilize the natural treatments noted in this section. Traditional treatment options for prostate cancer are divided into whether or not the cancer is confined to the prostate gland or has spread or metastasized to other areas of the body. When a cancer is confined to the gland, the new nerve-sparing total prostatectomy is often utilized to totally remove the prostate and its contained cancer from the body. There are, of course, many variables that enter into this decision, including the patient's age. The so-called radical prostatectomy offers a cure to most men whose cancer has not spread beyond the capsule of the prostate. Although there are potential side effects from this surgery—including impotency, incontinence, bleeding, and other problems—most can be managed medically.

Another option that is being used more and more is radiation therapy. This therapy uses high energy x-rays to kill prostate cancer cells. Irradiation comes from a machine outside the body (external radiation therapy) or from radioactive materials inserted into the prostate gland where the cancer cells are found (internal radiation therapy). Radiation treatments are used to kill cancer cells, but these treatments also can have side effects—many of which are similar to the surgical procedure. In advanced cases of prostate cancer in which the cancer has spread beyond the capsule of the prostate, hormonal intervention has been used to slow the growth of the cancer. The hormonal therapy also has its own set of side effects.

A DAILY SUPPLEMENT TO PREVENT PROSTATE CANCER

God has revealed many natural vitamins, antioxidants, minerals, and plant-derived chemicals that can protect men from prostate cancer. Though we should all strive to eat five to nine servings of fruits and vegetables daily, for many of us this is an area where we continually fall short. However, God's hand of protection has reached down and now given us the technology to extract multiple compounds from the plant and animal kingdom to help protect us from prostate and other cancers.

You should be on one of the current state-of-the-art, high-technology, daily supplements that incorporate not just the antioxidant vitamins and minerals, but also the various plant extracts such as sulforaphane from broccoli and cabbage, lycopene from tomatoes, and catechins from green-tea extracts. It is now possible for you to maintain steady blood levels of these substances by ingesting measured amounts daily with your supplement. (For information on our basic nutrient supplement which contains all of the previously-mentioned substances, see the Resources Available section at the end of this book.)

Chapter 4

PRAYING WITH UNDERSTANDING FOR PROSTATE DISEASE

Chapter 4

PRAYING WITH UNDERSTANDING FOR PROSTATE DISEASE

Up until now we have dealt mainly with the natural side of healing from prostate disease. Please don't misunderstand, however—prayer is the most important weapon we have against disease. In my twenty-five years of medical practice, I have found that combining the natural principles God gave us with the supernatural power of prayer is the most effective way to see healing manifest in our bodies. The moment you pray, healing begins in your body. The total healing manifestation may occur instantly or it may be a process over a period of time, which may be combined with things you might do in the natural such as outlined in this book.

To know what actions God desires you to take, you need to pray about prostate disease with understanding. The Bible urges us to pray with understanding: "What is it then? I will pray with the spirit, and I will *pray with the understanding* also" (1 Corinthians 14:15; emphasis mine). To pray with understanding, apply these six principles that will reveal your personal *Pathway to Healing*.

PRINCIPLE 1:
CAST YOUR CARES ON THE LORD

Negative, unhealthy, and destructive emotions like fear, anxiety, and worry can hinder your prayers about prostate disease and keep you from understanding what actions the Holy Spirit wants you to take. You cannot release your faith for healing until you have dealt with fear—fear will counter your faith. First Peter 5:7 AMP states, "Casting the whole of your care [all your anxieties, all your worries, all your concerns, once and for all] on Him, for He cares for you affectionately and cares about you watchfully."

If you are facing worries and fears about prostate disease, I want to reassure you that by the stripes of Jesus you have been healed (see 1 Peter 2:24). We often share with patients, "You must cast all of your anxieties and cares upon God. Cast your worries upon the Lord once and for all!"

I might have a patient worried about prostate disease pray these words:

Father, in the name of Jesus I come before Your throne. You instructed me in 1 Peter 5:7 to cast all of my care, all of my worry, and all of my anxiety once and for all upon You, and because You instructed me to do this, I know that I am capable of doing it and being set free of anxiety. So I cast the anxiety I have about prostate disease (cancer) upon You. You did not give me a spirit of fear, so I cast all of my concern about this problem upon You. I thank You

*that, according to Psalm 91:16, I will
be satisfied with long life. Amen.*

I will also warn a patient that fear may
well attack again in a day or so after we
have prayed. I then instruct him not to
pray this same prayer about fear again.
Instead, I explain that the enemy is
attacking the mind with fear and we
must now take authority over him:

*Satan, I have cast any anxiety about
prostate disease on my heavenly Father,
just as He told me to do. He would not
tell me to cast my cares upon Him
unless it was something I am capable
of doing. Therefore, I take authority
over you, Satan, and I command you
to stop attacking my mind with fear-
ful thoughts.*

PRINCIPLE 2:
PRAY AND PETITION GOD FOR
YOUR PATHWAY TO HEALING

Our key text here is Philippians 4:6-7, "But in every thing by prayer and supplication with thanksgiving let your requests be made known unto God. And the peace of God, which passeth all understanding, shall keep your hearts and minds through Christ Jesus." Pray according to these verses:

Father, I thank You that You will reveal to me the specific pathway that will lead to the healing of all symptoms related to my prostate. I thank You, Father, that in Jesus' name I will not experience problems any longer with this ailment, such as painful, difficult, and frequent urination, blood in my urine, pain in the pelvic area, and appetite and weight loss [list your specific symptoms].

I thank You, Father, that You have provided ways to protect my temple through the use of nutritional foods and natural supplements. They will protect me not only from the symptoms of prostate disease, but also from the increased risk of other infirmities that prostate disease can bring on.

Thank You, Father, that the answer to my prayer is on the way, in Jesus' name. Amen.

PRINCIPLE 3:
TEST YOUR OPTIONS
BY THE SPIRIT OF GOD

As you seek God for your *Pathway to Healing* for prostate disease, let the Holy

Spirit reveal your options, and check or stop any action that He does not desire you to take. The Bible instructs us: "And let the peace (soul harmony which comes) from Christ rule (act as umpire continually) in your hearts [deciding and settling with finality all questions that arise in your minds, in that peaceful state] to which as [members of Christ's] one body you were also called [to live]. And be thankful (appreciative), [giving praise to God always]" (Colossians 3:15 AMP).

The Spirit of God helps us to consider carefully our options—He umpires our choices—until we reach a decision that brings complete peace in our lives. Simply pray:

Father, I pray that the Holy Spirit will be an umpire in my life, guiding me to every right decision in Your will for me. Grant me Your peace in each decision that Your Spirit guides me through. In Jesus' name. Amen.

PRINCIPLE 4:
SPEAK TO THE MOUNTAIN

Now you are ready to speak to the mountain. Instead of just praying, petitioning, and testing, you can go even further in your walk with God. Jesus taught us to speak to our mountains and command illness to be removed.

"For verily I say unto you, That whosoever shall say unto this mountain, Be thou removed, and be thou cast into the sea; and shall not doubt in his heart, but shall believe that those things which he saith shall come to pass; he shall have whatsoever he saith" (Mark 11:23).

So when you speak to the mountain in prayer, you might say:

Father, I come before You in Jesus' name and I speak to that mountain called prostate disease (or cancer). I speak to my prostate gland and I command it to be normal, and I command my body and all the symptoms I have experienced to line up with the Word of God.

I speak to the painful, difficult, and frequent urination, blood in my urine, pain in my pelvic area, and appetite and weight loss [list your specific symptoms], *and command them to be gone. I speak to my entire body and command it to be free of all disease in the name of Jesus.*

Thank You, Father, that my sleep will be peaceful. I speak to my sleep and command it to be normal. I command my prostate function to be normal and my sleep to be uninterrupted by any untimely urgency.

Thank You, Father, for the power that You have given me through the name of Jesus to speak to my mountain. Thank You, Father, that through this authority I have dominion over the works of darkness that would attack my temple, which houses the precious treasure that You placed within me. In Jesus' name I pray. Amen.

PRINCIPLE 5:
PERSIST AND STAND FIRM
IN YOUR PATHWAY

When you have a revelation of God's *Pathway to Healing* prostate disease in your life, stand firm in what He is guiding you to do. "Wherefore take unto you the whole armour of God, that ye may be able to withstand in the evil day, and having done all, to stand" (Ephesians 6:13).

One way you stand firm and persist is to follow a proper nutrition and supplement plan to maintain prostate health in your body. Furthermore, you must persist in overcoming the annoying symptoms of painful, difficult, and frequent urination; blood in the urine; pain in the pelvic area; and appetite and weight loss (and others specific to you) while your prostate and immune system are being restored.

You must stand firm that as you do all that you can do in the natural to protect your temple through nutrition, exercise, and the use of natural supplements, you will not suffer the ravages of prostate disease.

PRINCIPLE 6:
MAINTAIN A FEISTY ATTITUDE AGAINST THE WORKS OF DARKNESS

In order to persist and stand firm, you must shift to a different attitude. Avoid the danger of becoming passive, giving up, or failing to fight this battle. Be feisty—even violent—in your persistence. "And from the days of John the

Baptist until now the kingdom of heaven suffereth violence, and the violent take it by force" (Matthew 11:12).

We encourage you to maintain a feisty attitude against all of the symptoms we have described that can take place in people's bodies with prostate disease. In other words, stand against painful, difficult, and frequent urination, blood in the urine, pain in the pelvic area, appetite and weight loss (and others specific to you), and all symptoms, which are works of the enemy.

As you follow God's *Pathway to Healing,* know that He wants you to be satisfied with long life. The word *satisfied* means that you are free of pain and symptoms in your physical body. We know that according to Revelation 22:2, "The leaves of the tree were for the healing of the nations." This scripture can have multiple meanings. One of the meanings is how God *did* work through natural substances found in plants to achieve our healing. God will give you clear direction as to what can be of particular help to your own body chemistry as you follow these specific principles. You will even be alerted to things that will not be helpful, or perhaps even harmful, to your body.

Chapter 5

YOUR NEXT STEPS
IN GOD'S PATHWAY
TO HEALING

Chapter 5

YOUR NEXT STEPS IN GOD'S PATHWAY TO HEALING

You have begun an important journey toward finding your *Pathway to Healing* prostate disease. Act on the truths you have received from God.

We want to review and summarize for you the steps you need to take now as you receive God's unique *Pathway to Healing* for you.

Step 1. Consult with a physician. Consultation with a physician can give you information about your body and give you particular insight as to how to pray for your symptoms. Even better is a Christian physician who will pray the prayer of agreement with you and give you all the facts known about your symptoms of prostate disease.

Step 2. Pray with understanding. Seek God in prayer and ask Him to reveal to you and to your doctor the best steps in the natural you can take in your *Pathway to Healing.*

Step 3. Ask the Holy Spirit to guide you to truth. Your doctor may advise you to have surgery, radiation, or use a prescription medication. You may feel led to use something natural such as saw palmetto. By referring to the information in this book, you can bring up the discussion of certain natural, plant-derived therapies that have been shown to help with prostate disease. Approach the physician by asking him if he would be willing to work with you and try the natural approach, or perhaps he would try the traditional approach in combination with the natural therapies we have discussed. I strongly encourage you to explore all the aspects of the pathway that we have shared with you—the pathway that God has created to strengthen and guard your body. Allow the Holy Spirit to guide you into all truth (see John 16:13).

Step 4. Maintain proper and healthy nutrition. Exercise and stay fit. We encourage you to adopt as many principles of the Mediterranean diet as possible and to incorporate into your daily diet the foods, herbs, and natural supplements we have discussed in this book to help your body overcome the symptoms you are battling.

Step 5. Stand firm in God's *Pathway to Healing* for you. Refuse to be discouraged or defeated. Be violently aggressive in prayer and in faith, claiming your healing in Jesus Christ.

We are praying that God will both reveal His *Pathway to Healing* prostate disease to you and give you the strength and faith to walk in it.

ENDNOTES

Chapter Two

[1] Patricia Nixon, PA-C. "New Clinical Trial of Medical Therapy for Benign Prostatic Hyperplasia." *Drug Benefit Trends.* 9, no. 3 (1997): 44-45. and James W. Cooper, Ph.D., and Robert W. Piepho, Ph.D. "Cost Effective Management of Benign Prostatic Hyperplasia." *Drug Benefit Trends.* 7, no. 8 (1995): 10-12, 15, 19-22, 32-33, 48.

[2] David W. Keetch, M.D. "Medical Therapy for Benign Prostatic Hyperplasia." *Infections in Urology.* 10, no. 2 (8 April 1997): 54-60.

[3] Timothy J. Wilt, M.D., M.P.H., Areef Ishani, M.D., Gerold Stark, M.D., et al. "Saw Palmetto Extracts for Treatment of Benign Prostatic Hyperplasia." *Journal of the American Medical Association* 280, no. 18 (11 November 1998): 1604-1609.

[4] R. Yasumoto, H. Kawanishi, T. Tsujuno, et al. "Clinical Evaluation of Long-term Treatment Using Cernilton Pollen Extract in Patients with Benign Prostatic Hyperplasia." *Clinical Therapeutics* 17 (January/February 1995): 82-87.

[5] Glen S. Gerber, Franklin C. Lowe, and Samuel Spigelman. Presentation at the 82nd

Annual Meeting of the Endocrine Society. Toronto, Canada: July 19-21, 2000.

Chapter Three

[1] American Cancer Society. "Estimated New Cancer Cases and Deaths by Sex for all Sites, United States, 2000." Accessed: August 18, 2000. http://www.cancer.org/statistics/cff2000/data/newCaseSex.html.

[2] Edward Giovannucci, Eric B. Rimm, Graham A. Colditz, et al. "A Prospective Study of Dietary Fat and Risk of Prostate Cancer." *Journal of the National Cancer Institute.* 85, no. 19 (6 October 1993): 1571-1579.

[3] Jennifer H. Cohen, Alan R. Kristal, and Janet L. Stanford. "Fruit and Vegetable Intakes and Prostate Cancer Risk." *Journal of the National Cancer Institute.* 92, no. 1 (5 January 2000): 61-68.

[4] Edward Giovannucci, Albert Ascherio, Eric B. Rimm, et al. "Intake of Cartenoids and Retinol in Relation to Risk of Prostate Cancer." *Journal of the National Cancer Institute.* 87, no. 23 (6 December 1995): 1767-1776.

[5] Robert S. DiPaola, M.D., Huayan Zhang, M.D., George H. Lambert, M.D., et al. "Clinical and Biological Activity of an Estrogenic Herbal Combination (PC-PES) in Prostate Cancer." *The New England Journal of Medicine.* 339, no. 12 (17 September 1998): 785-791.

REGINALD CHERRY, M.D.

A MEDICAL DOCTOR'S TESTIMONY

For six years of my life I lived in a dusty, rural town in the Ouachita Mountains of western Arkansas. In those childhood years, I had one seemingly impossible dream—to be a doctor! Through God's grace, I attended premed at Baylor University and graduated from The University of Texas Medical School in San Antonio, Texas. Throughout those years, I felt God tug on my heart a number of times, especially through

Billy Graham as he preached on television. But I never surrendered my life to Jesus Christ.

In those early years of practicing medicine, I met Dr. Kenneth Cooper and was trained in the field of preventive medicine. In the mid-seventies, I moved to Houston and established a medical practice for preventive medicine. Sadly, at that time money became a driving force in my life.

Nevertheless, God was good to me. He brought into our clinic a nurse who became a Spirit-filled Christian, and she began praying for me. In fact, she had her whole church praying for me!

In my search for fulfillment and meaning in life, I called out to God one night in late November of 1979 and prayed, "Jesus, I give You everything I own. I'm sorry for the life I've lived. I want to live for You the rest of my days. I give You my life." A doctor had been born again. Oh, and by the way, that beautiful nurse who had prayed for me and shared Jesus with me is now my wife, Linda!

Not only did Jesus transform my life; He also transformed my medical practice. God spoke to me and said, "I want you to establish a Christian clinic. From now on when you practice medicine, you will be *ministering* to patients." I began to pray for patients seeking God's *Pathway to Healing* in the supernatural realm as well as in the natural realm.

Over the years, we have witnessed how God has miraculously used both supernatural and natural pathways to heal our patients and to demonstrate His marvelous healing and saving power.

I know what God has done in my life, and I know what God has done in the lives of my patients. He can do the same in your life! He has a unique *Pathway to Healing* for you! He is the Lord that heals you (see Exodus 15:26), and by His stripes you were healed (see Isaiah 53:5).

Know that Linda and I are standing with you as you seek God's *Pathway to Healing* prostate disease.

If you do not know Jesus Christ as your personal Lord and Savior, I invite you to pray this prayer and ask Jesus into your life:

Lord Jesus, I invite You into my life as my Lord and Savior. I turn away from my past sins. I ask You to forgive me. Thank You for shedding Your blood on the cross to cleanse me from my sin and to bring healing to my body. I receive Your gift of everlasting life and surrender all to You. Thank You, Jesus, for saving me. Amen.

ABOUT THE AUTHOR

Reginald B. Cherry, M.D., did his premed at Baylor University, graduated from the University of Texas Medical School, and practiced diagnostic and preventive medicine for over twenty-five years. His work in medicine has been recognized and honored by the city of Houston and by Texas Governor George W. Bush. Dr. Cherry's wife, Linda, is a clinical nurse who has assisted Dr. Cherry with patients during these twenty-five years. Dr. Cherry and Linda also appear weekly on their television program, "The Doctor and the Word," which goes into more than 100 million households. Dr. Cherry speaks and lectures extensively and his first two books, *The Doctor and the Word* and *The Bible Cure,* have made the bestsellers' list. His latest book is entitled *Healing Prayer.* Dr. Cherry and Linda are now working full-time in Reginald B. Cherry Ministries to help people find their *Pathway to Healing* and to see the manifestation of their healing by combining the natural and the supernatural revelation and power God has given to them.

God's Pathway to Healing Prostate—
This minibook is packed with enlightening insights to men who are searching for ways to prevent prostate disease or who have actually been diagnosed with prostate enlargement or cancer. Discover how foods, plant-derived natural supplements, and a change in diet can be combined with prayer to help you find a *Pathway to Healing* for prostate disease.

$10.00 + S&H

Healing Prayer—A fascinating, in-depth look at a vital link between spiritual and physical healing. Dr. Cherry presents actual case histories of people healed through prayer, plus the latest information on herbs, vitamins, and supplements that promote vibrant health. This is sound information you need to keep yourself healthy—mind, soul, and body.

$19.99 + S&H

God's Pathway to Healing: Herbs That Heal—Learn the truth about common herbal remedies and discover the possible side effects of each. Discover which herbs can help treat symptoms of insomnia, arthritis, heart problems, asthma, and many other conditions. Read this minibook and see if herbs are part of God's *Pathway to Healing* for you.

$10.00 + S&H

God's Pathway to Healing Menopause— This minibook is full of helpful advice for women who are going through what can be a very stressful time of life. Find out what foods, supplements, and steps can be taken to find a *Pathway to Healing* for menopause and perimenopause.

$10.00 + S&H

The Bible Cure—(now in paperback) Dr. Cherry presents truths hidden in the Bible taken from ancient dietary health laws, how Jesus anointed natural substances to heal, and how to activate faith through prayer for health and healing. This book validates scientific medical research by proving God's original health plan.

$9.95 + S&H

The Doctor and the Word—(now in paperback) Dr. Cherry introduces how God has a *Pathway to Healing* for you. Jesus healed both instantaneously and supernaturally, while other healings involved a process. Discover how the manifestation of your healing can come about by seeking His ways.

$10.99 + S&H

Bound Volume of Study Guides—Receive thirty-five valuable resource study guides from topics Dr. Cherry has taught on television over the past fourteen years—cancer, vitamins, the immune system, weight loss, chronic fatigue, arthritis, nutrition, diabetes, and many other subjects.

$20.00 + S&H

Basic Nutrient Support—Dr. Cherry has developed a daily nutrient supplement that is the simplest to take and yet most complete supplement available today. Protect your body daily with natural substances that fight cancer, heart disease, and many other diseases. Call 1-800-339-5952 to place your order. Mention service code "K144" when ordering.

$49.95 + S&H

BECOME A *PATHWAY TO HEALING* PARTNER TODAY

We invite you to become a **Pathway Partner** of Dr. Cherry's ministry. We ask you to stand with us in prayer and financial support as we provide new programs, new resources, new books, minibooks, and a unique, one-of-a-kind monthly newsletter.

Our monthly *Pathway to Healing* **Partner Newsletter** is packed with medical and biblical information that only Pathway Partners receive. Here are the features our newsletter contains:

Fearfully & Wonderfully Made (Psalm 139:14)—Medical science is continually discovering what Scripture already reveals—that our bodies are miraculous creations given to us by God. In this feature, Dr. Cherry shares medical facts about our temples (how doctors diagnose thyroid disease by looking at the eyebrows, for example) and how God designed our immune system, hormones, arteries, kidneys, etc. to work in balance the way God "made" us.

Ask Dr. Cherry: Your Questions Are Answered (Luke 11:5-10)—Read Dr. Cherry's direct responses each month to your specific questions. He will provide you with both clear instruction and precise information by answering your questions (space permitting).

I Will Allow None of These Diseases on You (Exodus 15:26)—This monthly feature uncovers what the Bible teaches about God's healing at work in your temple and how God has provided protection for you from disease.

Praying With Understanding (1 Corinthians 14:15)—Dr. Cherry teaches you how to pray specifically for diseases, healing, and removing the mountain called disease from your life. There are prayers that Dr. Cherry and Linda have prayed personally with patients to remove their mountains of heart disease, cancer, diabetes, hypertension, arthritis, worry, depression, and other afflictions that attack our temples. The more you understand how to pray about a problem and how to speak to your mountain (Mark 11:23), the more effective your prayer will be (James 5:16).

Good Reports Give Happiness & Health (Proverbs 15:30)—We share good reports of healing from our partners of what God is doing to give you hope and show you God's way out of disease. The reports are intended to give all the glory to God. Be encouraged as you read what God is doing to "satisfy you with long life."

Nutrition & Your Health (Genesis 1:29)—God has created plants, herbs, minerals, and certain proteins for you to consume for energy and for strengthening your immune system, your arteries, and health and wholeness in your body.

Through proper nutrition, you can stay healthy! Learn what to eat, how to exercise, what supplements fight disease, and how to maintain a proper balance of nutrition in your *Pathway to Healing*.

Linda's Kitchen (Exodus 23:25)— Linda's recipes are filled with good nutrition and will teach you how to eat healthily, according to God's nutritional health laws. They are based on the wealth of knowledge gleaned from the Levitical dietary laws and wisdom revealed in Scripture about how to take care of our bodies. Read about how she cooks at home using her actual recipes.

In addition, we'll provide you with Dr. Cherry & Linda's ministry calendar, broadcast schedule, resources for better living, and special monthly offers.

Call or write to the address on the following page to obtain information on how you can receive this valuable information.

Pathway to Healing **Partner Newsletter**—Available to you as you partner with Dr. Cherry's ministry through prayer and monthly financial support to help expand this God-given ministry. Pray today about planting a seed in this unique ministry of healing and health. Contributions of $10.00 or more monthly will bring this valuable information into your home each month.

Become a Pathway Partner today by

writing:

Reginald B. Cherry Ministries, Inc.

P. O. Box 27711

Houston, Texas 77227

Visit our website:

www.drcherry.org

God's Pathway to Healing
Prostate

God's Pathway to Healing:
Herbs That Heal

God's Pathway to Healing
Menopause

Additional copies of this book
and other book titles
from ALBURY PUBLISHING are
available at your local bookstore.

ALBURY PUBLISHING
P. O. Box 470406
Tulsa, Oklahoma 74147-0406

For a complete list of our titles,
visit us at our website:

www.alburypublishing.com

For international and Canadian orders,
please contact:

Access Sales International

2448 East 81st Street

Suite 4900

Tulsa, Oklahoma 74137

Phone 918-523-5590

Fax 918-496-2822